On The Road

fitness, nutrition, +
100 motivational quotes
for the road

Robert B. Walker

I0039131

Copyright © 2019 by Robert B. Walker

All rights reserved. No part of this publication may be reproduced, stored in a retrieval system, or transmitted in any form or by any means — electronic, mechanical, photocopy, recording, or any other — except for brief quotation in printed reviews, without the prior written permission of the publisher.

Published by The Core Media Group, Inc., P.O. Box 2037, Indian Trail, NC 28079.

Cover & Interior Design: Ashlyn Helms

Printed in the United States of America.

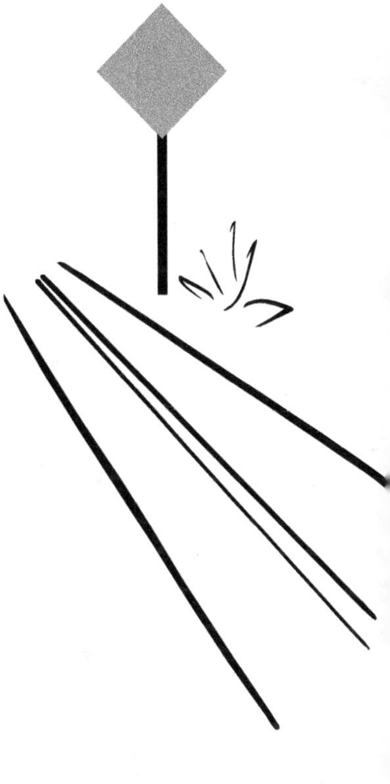

a note from the author

As I have traveled across the country every year, driving instead of flying, I have enjoyed seeing and experiencing all flavors of life. Each of these journeys have equipped me to write this book, and through this process I have learned to redeem and enjoy my time on the road.

During my idle time, I have found that investing in myself, through exercising and eating healthy, is more beneficial to me than scrolling through my phone. The goal is to make exercise a part of your state of mind. You can do these exercises anywhere and anytime, with your family or by yourself. Please do not attempt to do any of these exercises while your car is in motion. Finding healthy options on the go can be a constant challenge. I know that the nutrition section will be a benefit to your healthy lifestyle. The quotes I have written are designed to motivate, encourage, and inspire you on your life journey. Engage your mind and body, not just your gear, while you are on the road.

-Robert

roadmap

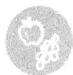

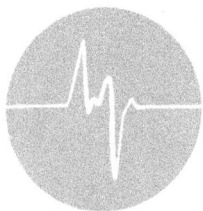

fitness

For videos of these exercises,
please visit our YouTube channel:

OnTheRoadFitness

in the car

FRONT ARM CURL

Hands in a fist, knuckles facing down.

Right Arm
Full Curl - 1 set of 10
Half Curl - 1 set of 10
Mini Curl - 1 set of 10

Left Arm
Full Curl - 1 set of 10
Half Curl - 1 set of 10
Mini Curl - 1 set of 10

TODAY'S MOTIVATION

**Building your own success is much more important
than someone handing you success.**

REVERSE CURL

Hands in a fist, knuckles facing up.

Right Arm
Full Curl - 1 set of 10
Half Curl - 1 set of 10
Mini Curl - 1 set of 10

Left Arm
Full Curl - 1 set of 10
Half Curl - 1 set of 10
Mini Curl - 1 set of 10

TODAY'S MOTIVATION

Never allow minor challenges to sidetrack your mental focus. Use the minor challenges to build the foundation of your mental strength.

HAMMER CURL

Hands in a fist

Right Arm (knuckles to the right)
Full Curl - 1 set of 10
Half Curl - 1 set of 10
Mini Curl - 1 set of 10

Left Arm (knuckles to the left)
Full Curl - 1 set of 10
Half Curl - 1 set of 10
Mini Curl - 1 set of 10

TODAY'S MOTIVATION

Work your wins into existence.

INSIDE CURL

With your hands in a fist, sweep your fist from your lap to your chest.

Right Arm - 1 set of 10

Left Arm - 1 set of 10

TODAY'S MOTIVATION

**Many people will say you cannot do it,
few will say you can.**

BENCH PRESS

With your hands in a fist, extend both arms out in front of you, and bring them back to your chest.

1 set of 10

TODAY'S MOTIVATION

**Extraordinary moments don't take place without
extraordinary preparation along the way.**

INCLINE CHEST PRESS

With your hands in a fist, push both arms out in an incline, and bring them back to your chest.

1 set of 10

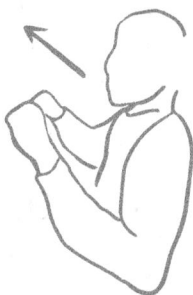

TODAY'S MOTIVATION

Your mindset can counter any setback.

MILITARY PRESS

With your hands in a fist, push both arms out over your head, and bring them back to your chest.

1 set of 10

TODAY'S MOTIVATION

**Maintain a high level of confidence in your skill set.
Never allow others to take what you already own. It is
your confidence, not theirs, so keep ownership of it.**

SHOULDER RAISES

Extend your arms straight out in front of you, with your hands in a fist. Lift your arms straight up.

Right Arm - 1 set of 10

Left Arm - 1 set of 10

Both Arms - 1 set of 10

TODAY'S MOTIVATION

Build up those who will continue your legacy.

SHOULDER SHRUGS

Lift your shoulders straight up toward your ears, then release your shoulders.

Right Shoulder - 1 set of 10

Left Shoulder - 1 set of 10

Both Shoulders - 1 set of 10

TODAY'S MOTIVATION

It is never too late to change how people perceive you.

SHOULDER HOLD

Lift your shoulders straight up toward your ears and hold for 3 seconds before releasing.

1 set of 10

TODAY'S MOTIVATION

**If who you are is not who you want to be, stop making
excuses, and start making an effort to become
that person.**

PECK DECK

With your hands in a fist and your arm in an upward 90-degree angle, sweep your arm inward towards your chest.

Right Arm - 1 set of 10

Left Arm - 1 set of 10

TODAY'S MOTIVATION

Invest your time with people who will cultivate growth in your life.

DOUBLE PECK DECK

With your hands in a fist and your arms in an upward 90-degree angle, sweep your arms inward towards your chest.

1 set of 10

TODAY'S MOTIVATION

**Passion will lead you to success.
Lack of passion leads you nowhere.
Bring passion for the work you love.**

PRAYING HANDS

Place your hands in a praying position under your chin. Chop down to a 90-degree angle.

1 set of 10

TODAY'S MOTIVATION

**This world is only hopeless when we refuse to be the
hope for others.**

HAND CIRCLES

With your hands in a fist, roll your hands one overtop of the other in a circular motion.

Forward - 1 set of 10

Backward - 1 set of 10

TODAY'S MOTIVATION

Life is full of curves, but it always straightens out.

DOUBLE BICEP

With your arms parallel to the ground outstretched, bend your arms towards your shoulders.

Full - 1 set of 10
1/2 - 1 set of 10
Mini - 1 set of 10

Hold for 2 sec. before releasing

TODAY'S MOTIVATION

Blessings come from sacrifice.

SHADOW BOX

With your hands in a fist, rapidly punch forward in front of your face.

10-15 seconds

TODAY'S MOTIVATION

**Let others see the fire in your eyes to be what you
were destined to become.**

STRESS SHAKE

Relax and loosen your hands by shaking them rapidly.

Towards the Right - 6 seconds

Towards the Left - 6 seconds

Upward - 6 seconds

TODAY'S MOTIVATION

**One of the most beautiful things in life is
the calm after the storm.**

CALF RAISES

Raise your heels up while keeping your toes on the ground.

1 set of 20

TODAY'S MOTIVATION

You will never be on top of the world if you aren't willing to make the climb.

LEG RAISES

Lift one leg up while keeping it in a 90-degree angle. Hold it for 3-10 seconds.

Right Leg - 1 set of 10

Left Leg - 1 set of 10

TODAY'S MOTIVATION

**Decide who you are, what you want to be known for,
and how you want to impact the world.**

DOUBLE LEG RAISES

Lift your legs up while keeping them in a 90-degree angle. Hold both legs up for 3-10 seconds.

1 set of 10

HOLD

TODAY'S MOTIVATION

**Don't be satisfied with mediocrity.
Find a way to excel.**

KNEE SQUEEZE

Push your knees together and hold them together for 10 seconds.

1 set of 6

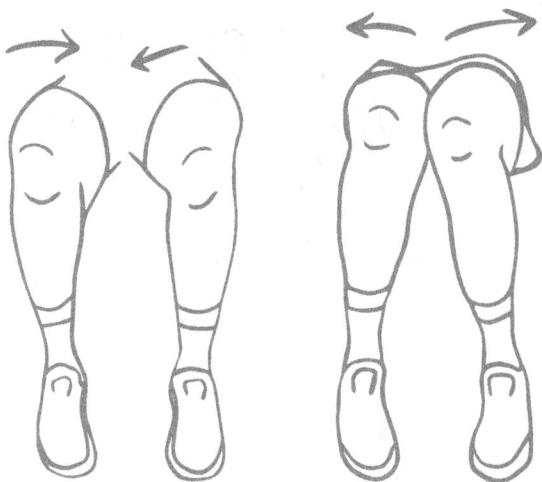

TODAY'S MOTIVATION

Being driven by a deep desire to be excellent and deeply thankful for the blessings in your life will jumpstart every day.

GLUT SQUEEZE

Tighten your gluts and hold them for 6 seconds.

1 set of 6

squeeze

TODAY'S MOTIVATION

Make the most of your time now.
We all will be replaced at some point.

SIT-UPS

Recline your seat back, and grab the steering wheel. Then, pull up and go back down.

3 sets of 10

This is a great exercise to do while you are waiting in your car for something or someone. Use your idle time.

TODAY'S MOTIVATION

**The sun rises every day. You, too, must rise every day.
Rise to the challenges that come with each day.**

BOUNCE

Rapidly bounce your legs while seated in your car.

30 seconds

TODAY'S MOTIVATION

Our desire for material things in life should not outweigh our appreciation for life.

outside of your car

CLEAN YOUR CAR

Get some exercise by cleaning all the trash out of your car.

TODAY'S MOTIVATION

**Before you weigh in, drop off your cares
and burdens into God's grace.
You will see your heart will be much lighter.**

WALK

Walk some laps around your car.

5 laps clockwise

5 laps counterclockwise

TODAY'S MOTIVATION

Never let someone walk away wondering if you truly care about them. Say it. Write it. Show it.

TOUCH TOES

To help stretch your body, bend down and touch your toes.

1 set of 3

Hold for 5 seconds when touching your toes

TODAY'S MOTIVATION

Comparing yourself to others limits what you can achieve.

REACH UP

To help stretch
your back,
lift your arms
straight up and
reach upwards.

10-15 seconds

TODAY'S MOTIVATION

**Rise to the occasion as a unit,
instead of as an individual.**

CALF STRETCH

Stand with the ball of your foot leaning up on a curb or step. With your heel on the ground, lean forward.

Right Calf - 10-15 seconds

Left Calf - 10-15 seconds

TODAY'S MOTIVATION

**Getting stronger does not always mean physically,
but rather mentally, emotionally, and spiritually.**

ARM CIRCLES

With both of your arms straight out, parallel to the ground, move your arms in a circular motion.

Forward - 20 seconds

Backward - 20 seconds

TODAY'S MOTIVATION

A comeback is dependent on you.

STRETCH

Stretch your body according to preference.

1 minute

STRETCH

TODAY'S MOTIVATION

There is a constant battle between freedom and control, but you cannot gain freedom without self-control.

STORE LAPS

Go into a store and do some laps. You could also do some laps outside of the store.

2-3 laps

REST STOP

TODAY'S MOTIVATION

**When you think the race is finished it is just beginning.
One victory does not mean the race of life is
completed. Keep pushing!**

PUSH-UPS

Get some old
gloves and do
some standing
push-ups
while you are
pumping gas.

15-20 push-ups

TODAY'S MOTIVATION

**To be outstanding, choose exceptional people to push
you toward your goals.**

JUMP-UPS

Extend your arms upward, reach and jump.

15-20 jump-ups

TODAY'S MOTIVATION

Breakaway from whatever it is that's keeping you from achieving your goals.

JUMP ROPE

Keep a jump rope in your car. Take it out at a rest stop and get some exercise.

10-20 jumps

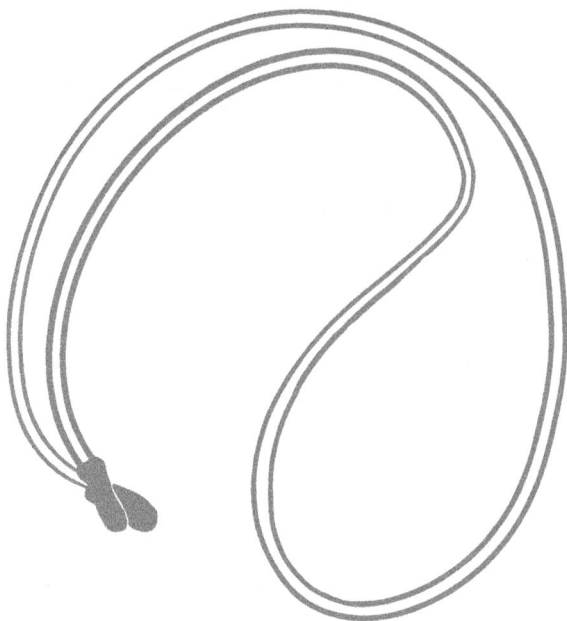

TODAY'S MOTIVATION

"Never let a day pass without taking a step toward your dreams. This is the only way they become reality."

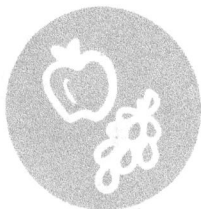

nutrition

breakfast

HARD BOILED EGGS

Where Do I Find It?

Grocery Stores

Prepare it at Home

Delis

Gas Station Markets

Convenience Stores

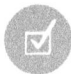

Benefits

Easy to Eat.

Keep you feeling full for longer periods of time.

Vitamins & Nutrients

5-7g of protein per egg

Choline - Helps improve brain function for faster reaction time

B12 - Helps oxygen uptake in cells for better performance and increased energy

Vitamin D - Improves bone strength

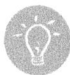

Tips

Add some salt for an extra flavor boost. It will also help replace the sodium lost when sweating to prevent cramping and dehydration.

OTR

INSTANT OATMEAL

Where Do I Find It?

Grocery Stores

Delis

Convenience Stores

Fast Food Restaurants

Diners

Benefits

High in carbohydrates and fiber.

Vitamins & Nutrients

Carbohydrates - Increase energy and refuel between active periods

Fiber - Helps digestion and increases fullness

B Vitamins - Help energy metabolism

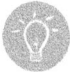

Tips

Look for whole grain oats. Eat it with hard boiled eggs, cheese, or add in nuts/peanut butter to stay full for a longer period of time.

OTR

MIXED FRUIT

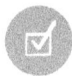

Where Do I Find It?

Grocery Stores

Delis

Convenience Stores

Some Fast Food Restaurants

Diners

Benefits

High in carbohydrates.

Easy to eat.

Refreshing.

Vitamins & Nutrients

Carbohydrates - Increase energy and refuel between active periods

Bananas have potassium that prevents muscle cramping and dehydration.

Watermelon is 90% water and high in potassium for hydration. It contains citrulline which helps blood flow.

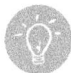

Tips

A tropical fruit such as a mango, pineapple, or banana is higher in sugar and carbohydrates. This makes them ideal to eat post workout.

Berries are lower in sugar but high in antioxidants to help your body repair faster. They are ideal to eat throughout the day.

OTR

GREEK YOGURT

Where Do I Find It?

Grocery Stores

Delis

Convenience Stores

**Some Fast Food Restaurants
(Look for a Yogurt Parfait)**

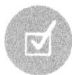

Benefits

Easy to eat on the go.

High in protein.

Vitamins & Nutrients

12-18g of protein per cup

Calcium - Helps with muscle contraction, bones, teeth, and hormone regulation

Probiotics - Improve digestion and gives you a healthier gut

Tips

Look for a low sugar yogurt.

Add your own fruit for extra nutrients and carbohydrates.

COTTAGE CHEESE

Where Do I Find It?

Grocery Stores

Delis

Convenience Stores

Benefits

Helps to regulate your blood pressure.

Helps to prevent osteoporosis.

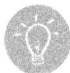

Vitamins & Nutrients

25g of protein per cup

High in casien protein, which is a slower digesting protein. It will keep your muscles anabolic overnight.

Calcium

Vitamin D

Tips

Add fruit for extra carbohydrates before or after your workout.

PROTEIN OATS

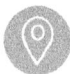

Where Do I Find It?

Make it at home and take it with you.

Benefits

Able to get a lot of calories out of it.

Can also be eaten as a day time or late night snack.

Vitamins & Nutrients

Carbohydrates - Increase energy and refuel between active periods

Fiber - Helps with digestion and increases fullness

B Vitamins - Help energy metabolism

Tips

Add honey to get extra carbohydrates.

Get creative with your protein powder flavor (fuels your muscles) and types of fruits (antioxidants).

Add collagen powder for strong soft tissue and joints.

GRANOLA & MILK

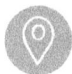 Where Do I Find It?

Grocery Stores

Delis

Convenience Stores

Diners

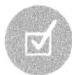 Benefits

Helps lower cholesterol.

Helps to prevent chronic diseases.

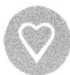

Vitamins & Nutrients

Carbohydrates - Increase energy and refuel between active periods

Fiber - Helps with digestion and increases fullness

Healthy Fats (if it contains nuts)

Vitamin D, Calcium, and Protein

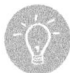

Tips

Add berries and nuts for extra nutrients and it helps you to feel full for a longer period of time.

snacks

STRING CHEESE

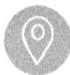

Where Do I Find It?

Grocery Stores

Delis

Convenience Stores

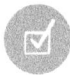

Benefits

Keeps you full by stabilizing your blood sugar.

Easy to eat on the go.

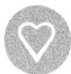

Vitamins & Nutrients

6g of protein

Calcium - Helps with muscle contraction, bones, teeth, and hormone regulation

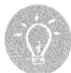

Tips

Pair this snack with some nuts for extra protein and fiber.

STICKS OF VEGGIES

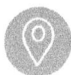

Where Do I Find It?

Grocery Stores

Delis

Convenience Stores

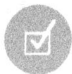

Benefits

Full of antioxidants and anti-inflammatory agents, which boost energy.

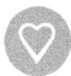

Vitamins & Nutrients

Micronutrients

Water - Most veggies are loaded with water, which helps hydration

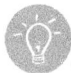

Tips

Add some peanut butter for extra protein and calories to stay full for a longer period of time.

JERKY

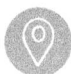

Where Do I Find It?

Grocery Stores

Delis

Convenience Stores

Gas Station Markets

Benefits

Rich in protein, but doesn't raise your insulin levels.

Easy to eat on the go.

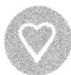

Vitamins & Nutrients

Protein

Sodium - Helps with hydration and prevents muscle cramping.

Iron

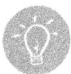

Tips

Look for natural jerky, which is nitrate-free.

NUTS AND SEEDS

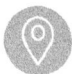

Where Do I Find It?

Grocery Stores

Delis

Convenience Stores

Gas Station Markets

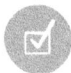

Benefits

Helps to reduce the risk of coronary heart disease.

Helps lower cholesterol.

 ## Vitamins & Nutrients

Protein and Fiber - Helps you to stay full for a longer period of time and aids in digestion.

Zinc - Post exercise muscle repair, neurotransmitter function for faster reaction time, and hormone regulator.

Choline

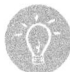 ## Tips

Add this snack to yogurt or cottage cheese.

Use this snack to make your own homemade trail mix.

QTR

DRIED FRUIT

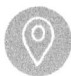

Where Do I Find It?

Grocery Stores

Delis

Convenience Stores

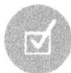

Benefits

Improves blood flow.

Reduces the risk of many diseases.

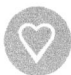

Vitamins & Nutrients

High in carbohydrates for post workout refueling.

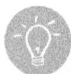

Tips

Eat this snack with some nuts to stabilize blood sugar and stay full for a longer period of time.

Create your own trail mix using this snack.

WHOLE FRUIT

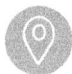

Where Do I Find It?

Grocery Stores

Delis

Convenience Stores

Some Fast Food Restaurants

Benefits

Refreshing.

Helps to lower your calorie intake.

Vitamins & Nutrients

Vitamin C

Potassium

Dietary Fiber

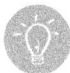

Tips

Add peanut butter for extra protein and calories to stay full for a longer period of time.

Add some salt for extra flavor. It also helps replace the sodium lost when sweating to prevent cramping and dehydration.

PROTEIN BARS

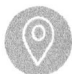

Where Do I Find It?

Grocery Stores

Convenience Stores

Gas Station Markets

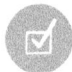

Benefits

Leaves you feeling full.

Easy to eat.

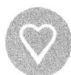 ## Vitamins & Nutrients

Carbohydrates

Protein

Healthy Fat

 ## Tips

Look for low sugar protein bars that contain at least 18g of protein, per bar.

CHOCOLATE MILK

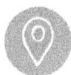

Where Do I Find It?

Grocery Stores

Convenience Stores

Gas Station Markets

Some Fast Food Restaurants

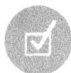

Benefits

Low cost replenishing option.

Fluid and electrolytes for hydration.

Vitamins & Nutrients

Great source of protein and carbohydrates

Calcium

Vitamin D

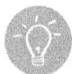

Tips

This is ideal for refueling post workout.

COCONUT WATER

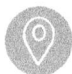

⊙ Where Do I Find It?

Grocery Stores

Convenience Stores

Gas Station Markets

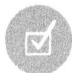

☑ Benefits

Natural sports drink.

Low in calories.

Natural electrolytes.

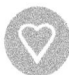

Vitamins & Nutrients

High in potassium for hydration

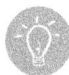

Tips

Add a pinch of salt for both potassium and sodium.

PRETZELS & HUMMUS

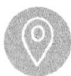

Where Do I Find It?

Grocery Stores

Convenience Stores

Gas Station Markets

Delis

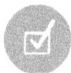

Benefits

Easy to eat on the go.

Packed with iron and vitamin C.

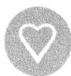

Vitamins & Nutrients

Carbohydrates from the pretzels

Sodium - Helps with hydration

Fiber from the chickpeas (in the hummus) helps with digestion and feeling full for a longer period of time.

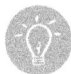

Tips

Try to avoid really salty pretzels.

QTR

PB & J SANDWICH

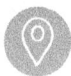

Where Do I Find It?

Grocery Stores

Convenience Stores

Delis

Pre-made and Pack

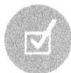

Benefits

Aids in digestion.

Helps to control cholesterol levels.

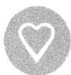

Vitamins & Nutrients

Fiber and carbohydrates from the whole grains

Carbohydrates from the jelly

Fiber and fat from the peanut butter

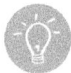

Tips

Instead of using whole grain bread, try eating this snack on crackers.

The combination of whole grains and nuts make this a complete protein. Pair it with some cheese for added protein. You can also add bananas for extra carbohydrates.

PICKLES OR OLIVES

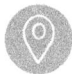

Where Do I Find It?

Grocery Stores

Convenience Stores

Delis

Benefits

Pickles - Help restless legs, and they are good for your eyes.

Olives - Help improve nerve function, and healthier hair growth.

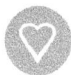

Vitamins & Nutrients

Loaded with sodium for hydration

Pickles are a prebiotic fiber that helps maintain a healthy gut.

Olives have antioxidants and healthy fats.

Tips

Many stores now sell mini packs of pickles and olives. They are perfect for eating on the go!

GUACAMOLE PACKS

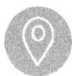

Where Do I Find It?

Grocery Stores

Convenience Stores

Delis

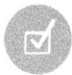

Benefits

Makes you feel full for a longer period of time.

Full of healthy fats.

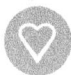

Vitamins & Nutrients

Loaded with healthy fat and fiber

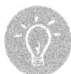

Tips

You can use these packets on your sandwich meat or dip veggies into them.

TUNA PACKETS

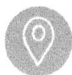 Where Do I Find It?

Grocery Stores

Convenience Stores

Delis

 Benefits

Good source of protein.

Vitamins & Nutrients

Protein

Omega 3 Fatty Acids

Sodium

Carbohydrates

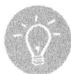

Tips

Vacuum sealed pouches have a fresher flavor and texture.

Pair this snack with some crackers for an extra crunch.

lunch/dinner

NITRATE-FREE MEAT

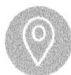

Where Do I Find It?

Grocery Stores

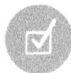

Benefits

Reduces the risk of cancer in the digestive tract.

 Vitamins & Nutrients

Protein

Sodium

Iron

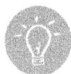 Tips

Make protein roll ups by wrapping the meat up in cheese.

OTR

GRILLED CHICK. SALAD

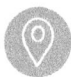

Where Do I Find It?

Grocery Stores

Delis

Convenience Stores

Fast Food Restaurants

Pre-made at Home

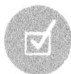

Benefits

Keeps you feeling lighter and more healthy.

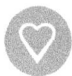 ## Vitamins & Nutrients

Protein

Fiber

Micronutrients

Iron

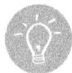 ## Tips

Add hard boiled eggs for extra protein.

Ask for double meat, if it is custom made.

For on-the-go, put your salad in a shaker bottle. Pour some dressing in it and shake it up!

SANDWICH WRAPS

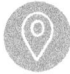

Where Do I Find It?

Grocery Stores

Delis

Convenience Stores

Some Fast Food Restaurants

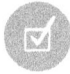

Benefits

Less calories than two pieces of bread.

Fast and easy to eat.

 ## Vitamins & Nutrients

Protein and Carbohydrates - Keep you full for a longer period of time

Iron

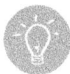 ## Tips

When creating or purchasing your sandwich wrap, avoid any fried meats and heavy sauces such as mayo or buffalo.

TURKEY/TUNA SAND.

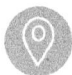

Where Do I Find It?

Grocery Stores

Delis

Convenience Stores

Some Fast Food Restaurants

Pre-made and Pack

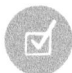

Benefits

Convenient.

Available almost anywhere.

Vitamins & Nutrients

Tuna - Omega 3 fatty acids to help prevent inflammation

Lunch Meat - Sodium and protein

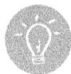

Tips

Add some pickles for sodium.

BURRITO BOWLS

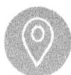

Where Do I Find It?

Fast Food Restaurants

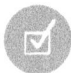

Benefits

Healthy balance of nutrients.

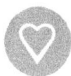

Vitamins & Nutrients

Great way to consume carbohydrates, protein and sodium

Prebiotic fiber from the sour cream helps to achieve a healthier gut.

Fiber and potassium from the guacamole.

Iron

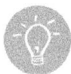

Tips

Ask for double meat to increase your protein intake.

If you are trying to maintain or lose weight, limit the amount of sour cream and guacamole.

TURKEY BURGERS

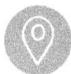

Where Do I Find It?

Some Fast Food Restaurants

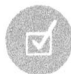

Benefits

Lower in calories and saturated fat than a traditional beef burger.

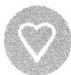 ## Vitamins & Nutrients

Protein and carbohydrates from lean meat

Iron

Choline

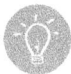 ## Tips

Try eating your turkey burger on a whole wheat bun.

GRILLED CHICK. SAND.

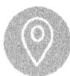

Where Do I Find It?

Delis

Fast Food Restaurants

Benefits

Good source of protein, vitamins, and minerals.

Uses less oil than fried meat.

Vitamins & Nutrients

Iron

Protein

Choline

Sodium

Carbohydrates (from the bun)

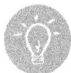

Tips

Always choose grilled meats over fried. Grilled meats prevent inflammation.

nutrients key

PROTEIN

Helps to

Build muscle

Prevent muscle breakdown

Found in

Meats - Fish

Dairy - Milk, Eggs, Yogurt

CARBOHYDRATES

Help to

Provide the body with energy
for athletic output

Refuel the body
after workouts

Provide the brain
with fuel

Found in

Grains - crackers, bread

Pasta

Fruits

Veggies

HEALTHY FATS

Help to	Found in
Improve hormone function	Avocado
Prevent inflammation	Fatty Fishes
Supply energy	Nuts/Nut Butter
Grow healthy skin	Cheese
	Olive Oil

CALCIUM

Helps to	Found in
Improve muscle contraction, strong bones (prevent injury), and strong teeth	Dairy
Regulate hormones	Dark Leafy Greens - Spinach, Kale, Collard Greens

POTASSIUM

Helps to

Maintain water balance in the cell (keep you hydrated)

Improve muscle contraction

Found in

Bananas

Avocado

Coconut

SODIUM

Helps to

Keep you hydrated

Improve muscle contraction

Balance fluid in the body

Found in

Jerky

Pickles

Lunch Meat

Chicken

VITAMIN D

Helps to	Found in
Build strong bones	Eggs
	Milk
	Cereal
	Salmon

CHOLINE

Helps to	Found in
Improve brain function (Faster reaction time & thinking)	Eggs
	Meat
Make faster muscle contractions	

ZINC

Helps to	Found in
Repair muscles after exercise	Meats
Improve neurotransmitter function	Nuts
Regulate hormones	

OMEGA 3 FATTY ACIDS

Help to	Found in
Prevent inflammation	Fatty Fishes - Tuna, Salmon, Mackerel
Prevent muscle loss	
Prevent DOMS (Post exercise muscle soreness)	

FIBER

Helps to	Found in
Keep your gut healthy	Avocado
Keep you full longer	Whole Grains
Produce healthy bowel movements	Veggies
	Fruit

PREBIOTIC FIBER

Helps to	Found in
Feed the probiotic fibers in your gut in order to have a healthy gut	Pickles
	Sour Cream
	Sauerkraut

ANTIOXIDANTS

Help to

Prevent cellular damage

Found in

Berries

Olives

Dark Leafy Greens

IRON

Helps to

Convert carbs during exercise

Bring oxygen to your blood

Improve proper muscle function

Found in

Chicken

Red Meat

Beans

Lentils

Leafy Greens

motivational quotes

Live in the now, not the
yesterday or tomorrow.
For the now is where you
are. Yesterday is gone,
and tomorrow is not here.
Let your purpose be about
making a difference today.

The quality of our
friendships determines the
values of our lives.

The difference between good and great is simple: sacrifice. Be up early, stay late, get your rest, then do the rest. It may not always feel the best, but it will be for the best.

―――――――

One of the least appreciated skills of successful people is their ability to choose quality friends.

You can borrow a suit, lease a car and rent a house. But you must own your character, and it will be defined by who you are and what you do.

———————————

Build bridges to people. This will allow you to construct relationships that have lasting value in your life.

If you gave others an all-access pass to your life, what would they find out about you? If there is something you don't want them to see, maybe you need to make a change for a better you.

Be the hope so that others may find their own.

A true friendship is born when two people decide that they're willing to be vulnerable.

———————————

So many people want love, yet so few are willing to put forth the effort to develop it. It takes hours of listening and encouraging others for love to flourish.

Never be the person who says, "I wish I would have worked harder, studied more, and spoken from my heart." Be the person who lives with passion and endurance.

———

Find the people who will tell you what you need to hear rather than what you want to hear. These are the people who love you with deep conviction and passion.

The people who go with you today may not be the people who need to go with you tomorrow. If they cannot grow with you, they should not go with you.

Live everyday prepared to say goodbye because one day you will.

In five years, if you find yourself still hanging around the same crowd, going to the same places, and speaking the same way, you may not be growing. The people you are with may be holding you back from your true potential.

Do not let where you come from keep you from getting where you want to go.

Laugh like a five-year-old.
Run like you are twelve.
Love with the passion of a
twenty-year-old. Think with
the wisdom of an eighty-
year-old.

Leadership can be very
lonely and frustrating.
Sometimes the decisions
you make will hurt others,
but you were chosen to lead.
Lead by being prayerful and
discerning.

Some people say, "I love you" with words but never with deeds. True love is a combination of the two.

———————

Learn how to appreciate the sacrifices that people make for you.

What is the destination
of your life? Draw a map
and layout your plan and
destination. You cannot get
to where you want to go if
you do not have a plan in
mind. Plan ahead to arrive
on time.

Smiling is the easiest way to
share the joy in your heart.

You can't change people, and you may not be able to change the world. However, you can change the people you let into your world and how you impact them.

―――――――――――

People are attracted to things that shine. Be the light and shine for all to see.

Every team is under construction daily. Be patient.

Perfection will always be paralyzing, and limit your potential, until you realize perfection is really pressing toward a goal that can only be chased and never caught.

To be aligned with your team means you must be totally committed to what is best for your team, not yourself.

———————————

You can prolong your career by putting the right people on your team.

Habits are hard to develop and break. Make your good habits a thing of the present and future, and make your bad habits a thing of the past.

The discipline of being a good team member is real work.

Doing the same things over and over again will result in a continuation of the past. If you don't want history to repeat itself, you have to adjust your game plan.

———————————

Forgiveness opens new doors in team relationships.

Building confidence is a
two-step process:
1-Stop thinking.
2-Start Believing.

Be thankful that you are
part of a team. You are part
of something greater than
yourself.

Whether you like your team or not, embrace each other's differences.

Courage is fear wrapped in the sweat of preparation.

Often times we wish we could retake our last shot and give it another try. The game is unforgiving, but that doesn't mean you have to be as well. Always give people a second chance.

Those who define greatness achieve greatness. If you cannot define greatness for your life, you cannot find it. Define greatness for yourself and you will find and achieve greatness.

Trophies all end up in
the attic. Enjoy your
achievements, but keep your
focus on the future.

———————————

Control your thoughts with a
winning attitude.

A good team will always say
it loved its coach and each
other. Breathe the right love
language into your team.

When you feel like your
hopes and dreams are
fading away just hang on!
That is a feeling not a fact!

Your skill set is an art, but
an artist who does not
perform may lose those
skills. Practice often.

———————————

What do you need to
sacrifice to achieve your
goals, dreams and vision for
your life?

Where you come from cannot hold you back from where you want to go, only you can.

———————————

Chase the money and lose the dream; chase the dream, and the money will come to you.

You cannot choose your teammates, but you can change their attitudes with encouragement and support.

———————————

To be a winner, surround yourself with winners.

Teach your team to play with the passion that fuels you.

What is behind me is done forever and cannot be changed. I am headed before me, toward my dreams and goals.

Love everyday. You never
know when you may lose
someone close to you.
Say, "I love you" more than
"Goodbye" or "Hello".

———————————————

Losses uncover your areas
of need. Embrace them.
Failure is a great teacher.

They say good things come to those who wait. I say good things come to those who work.

―――――――――――
―――――――――――

What value can you bring to the team besides your physical skills?

Believe First. Achieve second. To achieve you must always believe first. Do you believe?

Striving for excellence is important when achieving your goals. However, perfection is not realistic. Progress is realistic.

No matter what you think, we all started small. We only got here by growing.

———————————

Many times, to achieve our ultimate goals, God will break us only to remake us—to make our goals and dreams become reality.

If I told you that in order for you to reach your personal goals, you had to make one change in your life, could you or would you do this? If so, what are you waiting for? No one knows the future, but you can prepare now for your future and dreams by your choices.

If your goal is only to be better than the next guy, you are limiting yourself from what you can achieve.

Every day, do something
to take off and make your
dreams happen. If you
do nothing, nothing will
happen. Take off today.

Strive for the value you
leave, not the value you
take.

In order to be successful every day, you must do things that you don't enjoy doing. This will enable success, since you are willing to do the small things that no one sees.

———————————

People always say I want to be this or that, but they are never willing to make the commitment and sacrifice to attain those goals.

———————

Having a plan and implementing a plan are totally different. Take steps to implement your plan today.

OTR

Acknowledgments

I want to acknowledge and say thank you to all those that helped with this project:

Ashlyn Helms
Nadia Guy
Jevoni Robinson
Jaclyn Sklaver

All the people I have met on the road who have inspired me to write this book.

Additional Books by Robert B. Walker

Available in both digital and print versions.
To order the books below, visit www.thecoremediagroup.com

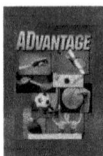

ADvantage: The Athletic Director's Ultimate Resource™

All the rules, regulations, policies, procedures, and forms an athletic director needs to operate an efficient and effective athletic program in a single, easily customizable source! You won't waste anymore time searching for the right form or procedures document. It's all right here, a wealth of information in one volume, and easily downloadable in a Microsoft Word format for you. Customize and duplicate as much as you need.

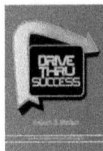

Drive Thru Success

What if finding success was as simple as ordering a combo at your favorite fast-food chain? In *Drive Thru Success*, author Robert B. Walker takes a refreshingly simple look at life as it relates to the drive-thru experience. Chapter after chapter, Walker's positive-thinking approach to the ups and downs of life will leave you ready to make the most of your own life, and perhaps a little hungry, too.

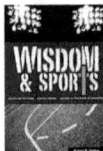

Wisdom & Sports

In *Wisdom & Sports*, verses from all 31 chapters of Proverbs are paired with spiritually encouraging stories of well-known athletes and thought-provoking devotionals. You will be inspired with these sports devotionals and sports stories.

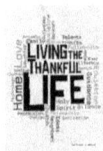

Living the Thankful Life

Living the Thankful Life includes 29 short stories about things Robert is thankful for. It also includes an area for you to write your own stories of thanks. Doing so enables you to create a legacy book for yourself, your family, and others about living a thankful life.

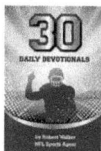

30 Daily Football Devotionals

30 Daily Football Devotionals contains 30 daily readings related to football. Each day contains a Bible verse and an inspirational story or thought to encourage you, both on and off the field. Included are areas for you to write notes or personal stories that you can reflect on throughout your athletic career.

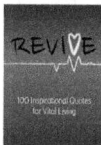

Revive: 100 Inspirational Quotes for Vital Living

Revive: 100 Inspirational Quotes for Vital Living is the first book to be released in the Revive series. It features 100 inspirational quotes on life, love, and personal relationships that are paired with relatable verses from the Bible. This book is a great resource for daily encouragement and for restoring vital energy and strength into your everyday life.

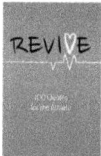

Revive: 100 Inspirational Quotes for the Athlete

Revive: 100 Inspirational Quotes for the Athlete is the second book to be released in the Revive series. It features 100 inspirational quotes for athletes on personal growth and sportsmanship. This book is a great resource for daily encouragement and will help you progress in your athletic life.

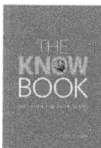

The Know Book

This life is filled with patterns—some obvious, some hidden. Whether we realize it or not, as we experience life-encountering situations, building relationships, making connections—we learn more and more about these rhythms of human existence. The question isn't whether or not these patterns exist. The important question to ask yourself is, "How much do I know?" Through fifty-two easily digestible chapters, *The Know Book* breaks down these themes of life and provides a guide for navigating through them. You've had the experiences, the relationships, and the personal convictions. Here's your chance to rediscover what you've known all along.

CHECK OUT

THE PRAYING ATHLETE™
QUOTE BOOK SERIES

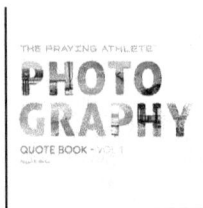

VOL. 1

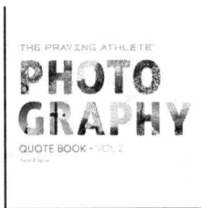

VOL. 2

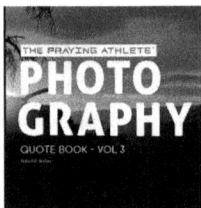

VOL. 3

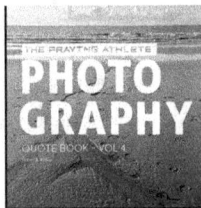

VOL. 4

The Praying Athlete Photography Quote Books celebrate God's glory and magnificence through His creation. They contain photos taken by Robert B. Walker, paired with his words of wisdom, motivation, and inspiration.

FOR MORE INFO AND MERCHANDISE, PLEASE VISIT
WWW.THEPRAYINGATHLETE.COM

The Praying Athlete logo

THE PRAYING ATHLETE QUOTE BOOK	THE PRAYING ATHLETE QUOTE BOOK	THE PRAYING ATHLETE QUOTE BOOK	THE PRAYING ATHLETE QUOTE BOOK
PLAYING THE GAME — VOL 1	TEAM — VOL 2	GROWTH & PREPARATION FOR THE FUTURE — VOL 3	KEEPING THE RIGHT MENTALITY — VOL 4
STAYING — VOL 5	PERSONAL — VOL 6	LIVING LIFE — VOL 7	LIVING LIFE — VOL 8

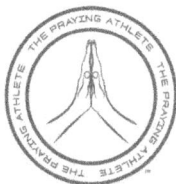

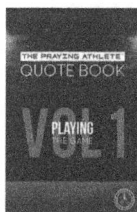

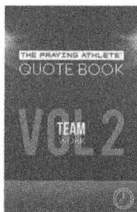

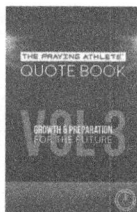

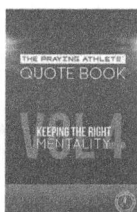

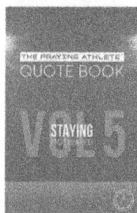

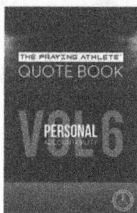

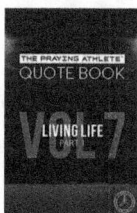

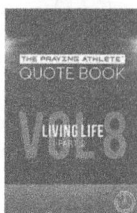

Our first eight volumes of *The Praying Athlete Quote Book* address numerous topics including, playing the game, teamwork, growth & preparation for the future, keeping the right mentality, staying motivated, personal accountability, and living life. Quotes and thoughts from Robert B. Walker, paired with Scripture from God's Word, give encouragement to each and every reader to be the best person he or she can be.

www.ingramcontent.com/pod-product-compliance
Lightning Source LLC
Chambersburg PA
CBHW060848280326
41934CB00007B/969

9 781950 465293